WARNING SIGNS OF KIDNEY PROBLEMS.

It is essential to know these signs.

By

Dr. DOUGLAS JASON

TABLE OF CONTENTS

ABOUT THE AUTHOR

INTRODUCTION

TABLE OF CONTENTS

WARNING SIGNS OF KIDNEY PROBLEMS.

It Is essential to know these signs.

INTRODUCTION

CHAPTER 1
ALWAYS FEELING TIRED

CHAPTER 2
RUDE SLEEP

CHAPTER 3
SKIN ITCHINESS

CHAPTER 4
SWOLLEN FACE AND FEET

CHAPTER 5
MUSCLE CRAMPS.

CHAPTER 6
Breathlessness

CHAPTER 7
FOGGY HEAD

CHAPTER 8

LOW APPETITE AND BAD BREATH

CHAPTER 9
FOAMY BROWN OR BLOODY URINE

CONCLUSION

ABOUT THE AUTHOR

Dr. DOUGLAS JASON is a certified dietician who has a strong passion for wellness and a big eagerness to help people all over the world. He uses healthy food, herbs, sauce, and other useful tools to help mankind realize its overall goal of optimum health.

INTRODUCTION

The kidneys are extraordinary organs that are essential to preserving our general health. They generate hormones that encourage the creation of red blood cells, filter waste materials, maintain fluid balance, and control blood pressure. However, kidney problems might occur, so it's important to be aware of the symptoms that point to possible difficulties. Early detection of these symptoms may help with quick diagnosis and treatment, which helps to avoid additional consequences. This writing will discuss some typical kidney disease warning signals, enabling readers to take preventative action for kidney health.

CHAPTER 1

ALWAYS FEELING TIRED

Your kidneys extract trash from your blood and excrete it in your urination. Poisons might accumulate when your kidneys aren't behaving adequately. Deficiency is a regular warning sign. You can experience fatigue, shortcoming, or problem-focusing. A hormone produced by the kidneys advises the body to create red blood cells. Your blood cannot nourish your muscles and brain with the essential quantity of oxygen if you have fewer of them.

CHAPTER 2

RUDE SLEEP

Studies suggest a connection between chronic kidney disease (CKD), which over time destroys your organs and may result in renal failure, and bedtime apnea. Because sleep apnea limits the amount of oxygen your body accepts, it may be toxic to your kidneys. Because of the constriction of the neck, toxicity expansion, and other factors, CKD may result in sleep apnea.

CHAPTER 3

SKIN ITCHINESS

This could happen if toxins assemble in your blood because your kidneys are unfit to remove them. This could result in inflammation or severe itching. Your kidneys could become less effective at balancing the minerals and nutrients in your body over time. Your skin may become parched and prickling as a result of mineral and bone infections.

CHAPTER 4

SWOLLEN FACE AND FEET

Liquids accumulate in your body as your kidneys battle to properly eradicate salt. This could result in swollen hands, feet, ankles, legs, or even the face. Your feet and ankles may notably show signs of edema. Additionally, the area surrounding your eyes may seem puffy if the protein is spilling out into your urine.

CHAPTER 5

MUSCLE CRAMPS.

Leg twitches as well as other kinds of pain may imply a kidney problem. Your muscles and nerves might encounter problems if the levels of sodium, calcium, potassium, or other electrolytes are out of balance.

CHAPTER 6

Breathlessness

A hormone called erythropoietin isn't produced by your organs in sufficient amounts when you have kidney disease. Your body's hormones tell it to begin eliciting red blood cells. Without it, you risk developing anemia and becoming breathless. Fluid proliferation is another factor. It could be tough for you to breathe. In extreme conditions, laying down could cause you to feel as if you're drowning.

CHAPTER 7

FOGGY HEAD

Toxins may harm your brain when your kidneys are unable to completely remove waste from your body. The oxygen your brain requires might be obstructed by anemia. You could have lightheadedness and memory and attention problems. Even basic things may become challenging for you if you get too confused.

CHAPTER 8

LOW APPETITE AND BAD BREATH

Your stomach may feel queasy or troubled due to a kidney infection. You may not have much of a food appetite as a result. That may sometimes result in weight reduction.

Uremia, a disease that formulates when your kidneys are incapable to filter out waste, may result. That could give your mouth a bad odor. Additionally, meals may taste metallic or odd if you have toxins in your system.

CHAPTER 9

FOAMY BROWN OR BLOODY URINE

Overproduction of the albumin protein may result in bubbly urination. That may be the outcome of renal problems. So too may be extraordinarily light or dark urine. Incorrect kidney function may also cause blood to enter your bladder. Kidney stones, tumors, or an infection are some conditions that may result in blood in the urine.

CONCLUSION

In conclusion, preserving optimum health and halting the spread of kidney disorders depend on being aware of the warning signals of renal issues. Individuals may seek prompt medical attention and get essential therapy and care by being aware of signs such as altered urination, edema, exhaustion, and chronic discomfort. A healthy lifestyle that incorporates regular exercise, a balanced diet, and drinking enough water may also have a big impact on kidney function. Remember, successful kidney disease management depends on early identification and action. By being aware and proactive, we can protect our kidneys and advance general well-being.